... .Wimpy to Winning

From Wimpy to Winning

The Young Athlete's Guide to Eating and Exercising

for Health, Energy, and Endurance

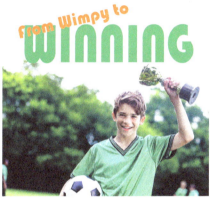

Karen R. Meyer

ISBN 978-0-692-95963-3

Copyright 2017 by Karen R. Meyer

Cover design by Janet Clark Shay, Cover photo © Steve Debenport/iStockphoto.com, illustrations, Karen Meyer

A note to parents

Parents, **you** are the key to helping your child get fit and active. Doctors agree that *many diseases begin in childhood*. Dr. Kenneth Cooper, the Air Force doctor who popularized aerobic exercising, warns, "Millions of our children–the majority of them in middle- and upper-middle-class homes–face the prospect of serious disease and shortened life spans because of **sedentary living** and **poor nutrition.**"

Educate yourself to help your family toward a lifetime of good health.

Contents

1. Are You Wimpy?

SOMETIMES WE ALL FEEL THIS WAY!

Rocky did, so he took charge and changed.

He realized his love of sweets was catching up with him when he tried out for the basketball team. He had

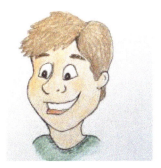

Hi! I'm Rocky.

trouble keeping up, partly because of the extra 25 pounds he wore around his middle like a donut. Coach took him aside and suggested he should cut out the sweet stuff and learn what to eat in its place.

Rocky will share some of the things he learned. Now he's the team captain, encouraging others to make good food choices so the team can play to its potential.

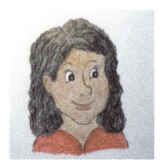

Hi, I'm Roxy

Roxy plays soccer. As a defender, she runs most of each game. By the second half, she would be really tired. She felt **WIMPY**.

The other teams took advantage of this, often winning because Roxy and her team couldn't keep up.

Roxy's coach gave her lots of good advice, both training exercises and diet changes. She will share some of the things she learned. Roxy is now the key to her team's defense this year.

DID YOU KNOW–The human body is the most complicated machine in the world.

Amazing facts

- Your body has 60,000 miles of blood vessels

- You use 200 muscles to take a single step

- Messages from your brain travel along your nerves at 170 miles per hour.

- Your femur (thigh bone) can support thirty times the weight of your body.

- The human heart pumps 45 million gallons of blood around the body in an average lifetime.

- Your body has enough iron in it to make a three inch nail.

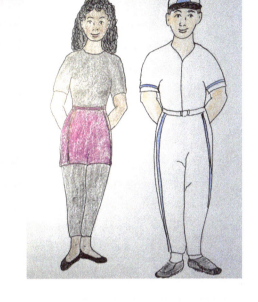

Your body is priceless.

This **valuable gift** is worth taking good care of.

We are *stewards* or caretakers of this gift, since it is on loan to us from God.

> **I Corinthians 6:20   Therefore, glorify God in your body.**

God hands out our bodies with different strengths and weaknesses,

but he has one *unbreakable rule: only one body per customer.*

Start today to take care of the body you have.

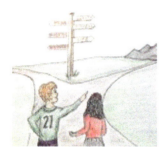

- **Regular daily exercise** is part of taking care of your body.

  The **muscles you use** get stronger.

  The muscles you ignore get weaker.

- **Choosing healthful food** is also important for your fitness, today and for the future.

Making choices for good health

The decisions you make today for your **million–dollar body** will affect your future. Today you are young and strong. You can't always be young, but you can keep your body strong. This book will help you choose wisely how to *EXERCISE* and **FUEL** your body.

Proverbs 10:17 Whoever heeds instruction is on the path to life.

WRITE YOUR GOALS

Skills you already have:

Skills you want to gain:

Long-term goals:

Staying Healthy

"Of the ten leading causes of death in America, five–atherosclerosis, stroke, heart disease, diabetes, and cancer–can be caused by a bad diet."[1]

Begin today to **make good health your goal**, and eating right and exercise as an enjoyable way to achieve it.

A note to young readers

You will find more new ideas than you can use at once! Highlight or underline some for trying out later. Add more cartoons in the blank spaces. Try out a new recipe. Jot down your own ideas.

1. Schwartzenegger, p. 42.

2. Feeding Your Body

FEEDING YOUR BODY

Food! We love to eat. Sometimes we will try new foods, but most of us stick with what is familiar. Perhaps the food you've always eaten is not the best fuel for your growing body, with the extra demands of a sport.

Be smart and learn which kinds of food your body needs to perform at the top level.

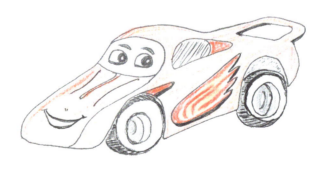

Ali, the race car.

Think of your body as a **finely tuned race car.** A race car's many systems work together to reach a high speed. The combustion system, braking system, electrical system, hydraulic system, and cooling system need specific fluids or equipment to work correctly.

BODY SYSTEMS

As an athlete, you "fuel up" your *body systems* every day with the foods you eat. Each system needs specific vitamins and minerals. Much of our food today comes from a factory instead of being grown by a farmer. The snacks, cereal, bread, and desserts you eat have been engineered to taste good, but contain fewer vitamins and minerals.

Choose a variety of fresh, simple foods, so your body gets all the nutrients you need.

Your body's ten main systems

1. muscular/skeletal system
2. urinary system
3. cardiovascular system
4. digestive system
5. endocrine system
6. reproductive system
7. respiratory system
8. lymphatic/immune system
9. integumentary system
10. nervous system

> ## Can you match the body systems with their description?

- A. sexual organs
- B. brain and nerves
- C. skin
- D. muscles and bones
- E. lungs
- F. glands producing hormones
- G. mouth, stomach, intestines
- H. excretes waste via urine
- I. heart, circulates blood
- J. organs protecting the body from disease
- Answers   1.-d 2.-h 3.-i 4.-g 5.-f. 6.-a 7.-e. 8.-j 9.-c 10.-b

These complicated systems **work together**, so you must keep all of them strong. For example, calcium , magnesium, and vitamin D are needed to keep your bones strong. Strong bones pair with strong muscles. Keep your muscles strong by eating foods rich in magnesium and calcium, and protein foods for repair.

A CHAIN IS ONLY AS STRONG AS ITS WEAKEST LINK

Give your body *all the nutrients* it needs to strengthen each of your body's ten systems. Then your strong body will be ready to compete.

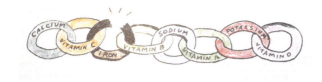

One broken link weakens the action of the rest

VITAMINS AND MINERALS

Of course you can name the six main vitamins. (A,B,C,D,E, and K)

Where are the vitamins hiding?

- Vitamin A   Green leafy vegetables, carrots, fruits, eggs

- B Vitamins   Whole grains, protein foods, fruits, vegetables, legumes

- Vitamin C   Fruits and vegetables

- Vitamin D   Milk and fish

- Vitamin E   Eggs, nuts and seeds, green leafy vegetables, and whole grains

- Vitamin K   Produced by the "good bacteria" in your gut, if you have not taken antibiotics. Restock good bacteria with yogurt and sauerkraut.

How many of the nine main minerals your body needs can you name? 1._____

2._____3._____

4._____5._____

6._____7._____

8._____9._____

Where are the minerals found?

- Iron   Meats, poultry, eggs, nuts, green leafy vegetables, fruits

- Calcium   Salmon, green leafy vegetables, broccoli

- Magnesium   Fruits, grains, green leafy vegetables

- Phosphorus   Meats, poultry, fish, nuts

- Potassium   Fruits and vegetables

- Copper   Meats, shellfish, nuts

- Selenium   Whole grains, fish, eggs

- Zinc   Shellfish, meats, whole grains, vegetables

- Trace minerals   Seafoods, green leafy vegetables

MEET THE NEEDS OF EVERY SYSTEM

- Your body is a complicated machine. Scientists, doctors, and nutritionists are finding surprising ways the nutrients in food work together in your body.

- **How can you make sure your body's needs are met by the foods you choose?**

- **Choose answer #1, #2, or #3 from the list below.**

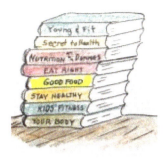

Learn lots of nutrition facts
from these books

#1. Read a stack of books on nutrition.

#2. Earn a college degree in nutrition.

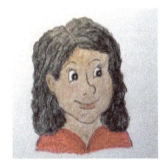

Roxy says, choose #3

#3. Eat a variety of high-quality foods from all six food groups.

WHAT IS A HIGH-QUALITY FOOD?

Look at the list of **Super Foods** in chapter five. These foods have *"high nutrient density."* That means they provide the protein or carbohydrates or other *macro*nutrients your body needs, AND they're packed with vitamins and minerals, the *micro*nutrients.

THE SIX MAJOR FOOD GROUPS

Are you in a food rut? Try to eat from **all six** food groups every day.

1. **VEGETABLES** All vegetables provide carbohydrates. Dark green leafy ones and orange ones have the most vitamins.
2. **FRUITS** Fruits are a good source of carbohydrates. Dark blue and purple ones are especially good for you.
3. **DAIRY** Dairy products have lots of calcium and vitamin D.
4. **MEATS AND SEAFOODS** Meat and seafood provide protein, the building block of the body. About 25% of your calories should come from protein.
5. **WHOLE GRAIN** Whole grains provide carbohydrates and the vitamins to process them into energy.
6. **NUTS, SEEDS, OILS** Nuts and seeds contain fat, a key ingredient for many body systems. Fat provides long-lasting energy and is needed for the body to absorb certain vitamins.

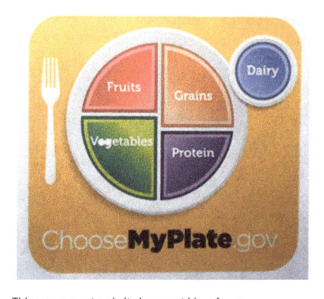

This government website has great ideas for you

The U.S. government website **<choosemyplate.gov>** has much helpful information on what to eat. Get on their email list to find out more about eating healthy foods every day.

The website's icon shows the main food groups and how much of each you should eat each day. (oils/fats are not shown, since they occur in several of the food groups.)

> **So, whether you eat or drink, or whatever you do, do all to the glory of God.   I Corinthians 10:31**

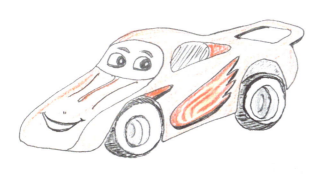

Ali is all fueled up

CARBOHYDRATES

Get Ready…   Your "race car" body is at the starting line. Are you all fueled up? Participating in sports puts high demands on your body. Playing a sport uses all your available energy. **Where does the energy come from?**

CARBOHYDRATES ARE THE MAIN SOURCE OF ENERGY FOR ATHLETES.

Carbohydrates are found mainly in grains, fruits, vegetables, and dairy foods.

WHICH CARBS SHOULD YOU CHOOSE FOR FUEL?

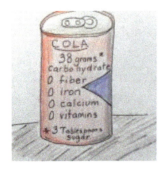

A soda–LQ or HQ?

Will you choose wisely? LQ carbs or HQ carbs?

Low-quality carbs These are the "junk foods" that you crave. They don't give you all the vitamins and minerals your body needs. They are changed rapidly into **energy**, but that's followed by a **drop in energy**, and fatigue sets in. They steal vitamins from your body.

So grabbing a candy bar is not the best option to get your energy/fuel. Filling up on **LQ** carbs means you are missing some of the nutrients your body needs.

Choose HQ carbs

High-quality carbohydrate sources include fruits, whole-grain bread, beans, vegetables, and milk. Because the carbohydrates in these foods are mixed with fiber and fat, their fuel is *metabolized* more slowly into your system and lasts longer. Metabolizing your food means it is chemically changed into a form your body can use for energy.

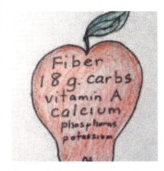

An apple has 18 grams of carbs, plus vitamins and minerals

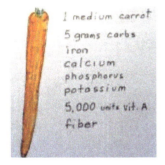

Carrots have fiber, carbs, vitamins and minerals

You need carbs

1. for energy before a game
2. to restock energy stores
3. for repair of tissue damage
4. for growth

Elite Kenyan Runners

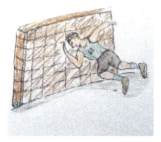

This runner "hit the wall"

- Elite Kenyan runners have a diet very high in carbohydrates. Seventy-six percent of their calories are from carbs. Most coaches suggest 50-60%. When other runners "hit the wall," (ran completely out of energy), those on a high-carb diet continued their pace. They ran 13% faster than those on a lower-carb diet.[1]

Sports Nutrition Chart

Calculate your carb needs to match your activity level.[2]

- **Mildly active...**(less than an hour of exercise), daily intake of 2.25-3. grams carbs per pound of body weight.

- **More active...** (an hour of exercise), daily intake of 3. -4.5 grams of carbs per pound of body weight.

- **Very active** (two + hours of exercise) 4.5-5.5 grams of carbs per pound of body weight.

- **For example**, a 100 lb. athlete who exercises for an hour a day will need to refuel on carbs by eating 300 to 450 grams of carbohydrates.

How Many Carbs are in Common Foods?

- Carbohydrates are weighed in **grams** for most charts; thirty grams is about an ounce. Look for online charts, but here are examples to get you started.
- A large banana has thirty grams of carbs.
- two slices of bread have thirty grams of carbs.
- one cup of spaghetti with meat sauce has thirty-five grams of carbs.
- ten ounces of milk has fifteen grams of carbs.
- two cups of popcorn with oil and salt has twenty grams of carbs.
- one medium apple, raw, has eighteen grams of carbs.
- one cup carrot, raw or cooked has ten grams of carbs.

WATER

Your body is about 60% water.

"Water is to your body what oil is to your car." No driver can go far without oil, and you will have many problems if you let yourself get dehydrated.

To perform at its best, your body must have water. Water lubricates your joints and other parts, keeps you cool, and helps rid the body of waste. **Water gives you** *energy.*

When you exercise, you perspire. **Don't wait until you're thirsty** to drink the water your body needs, since by that time you're already 1% dehydrated.

Key Takeaway

*For best performance, hydrate **before, during, and after exercise**. Keep the water bottle with you and keep drinking every chance you get.*

WHAT SHOULD YOU CHOOSE FOR YOUR DRINK?

Choose wisely.

- Water is the best drink, since it is absorbed fastest. Special athletic drinks slow absorption.[3]

- During exercise, add a small amount of carbohydrate (6-8%) to extend your endurance time. Make your own "sports drink" by flavoring your water with fruit juice.

- After exercise, drink a lot, but not all at once. Most athletes fail to rehydrate enough.

- **Avoid** diet sodas, commercial sports drinks,and fruit drinks with added sugar, high fructose corn syrup, or artificial sweeteners.

WHEN TO FUEL UP AND HYDRATE

TIMING FOOD AND WATER INTAKE BEFORE, DURING, AND AFTER EXERCISE

- Two hours **before exercise** eat a meal high in carbs, low in fat. Don't eat immediately before the event, since you'll divert energy to digestion. Hydrate well.

- **During exercise**, never wait for the "I'm thirsty" signal. Hydrate ahead *and* during exercise, by sipping.

- To avoid stomach and intestinal problems, avoid solid foods or high-carb drinks (over 8%) **during exercise**.

- **After an event**, replenish liquids by sipping (rather than drinking large amounts).

- **After an event**, eat high carbohydrate meals to replenish the energy you used up during exercise.**Avoid** "energy drinks" and anything else with caffeine, since caffeine is a diuretic. (Promotes urination). (Tea, coffee, many sodas, and chocolate all contain caffeine.)

CARBOHYDRATE LOADING BEFORE AN EVENT

Carbohydrate loading is a method some athletes use to make sure their muscles have stored as much energy as possible before a big competition.

- Begin a week before the event and gradually increase carbohydrate and fluid intake.

- Start the week with a heavy workout, emphasizing your weak areas.

- Taper the exercise downward each day.

- This makes seven days of *increasing* carb and fluid intake, matching seven days of *decreasing* the duration of the workouts.

EATING TO GAIN MUSCLE WEIGHT

- Both protein and carbohydrates are needed to gain muscle weight.

- About 350 extra calories per day are needed to gain a pound per week.

EAT TO PROMOTE ENDURANCE

- Some athletes run out of energy before the game is over. Don't let that happen to you!

- *Foods high in B vitamins* help combat fatigue. (Whole grains, meat, fish, eggs, and dairy products).

- *Low-quality carbs*, like donuts and cookies, are metabolized quickly, giving you a sugar high, followed by a dramatic drop in blood sugar level. **Low blood sugar means fatigue.**

- *Complex carbs** keep your energy level high to the end of the game or the race. Whole grains, fruits, and vegetables will give you the edge. *A carbohydrate is complex when it has the fiber and fat that came with it originally. Examples: whole grain vs. white flour, an apple vs. apple juice.

THE WRONG WAY TO GAIN TOP PERFORMANCE

***Anabolic steroids** are promoted as a way to build your muscle strength and endurance. These may instead cause damage to a healthy body. Many sports have banned the use of steroids, and they are **illegal without a prescription.**

*Other products are advertised to help athletes perform better, such as **caffeine drinks, energy bars, and herbal supplements**. Stick to the safe and healthy way to perform at your best–*eating healthful foods and practicing your skills.*

EAT TO PROMOTE OVERALL FITNESS

- Are you eating **real food** or

- products with **many artificial ingredients?**

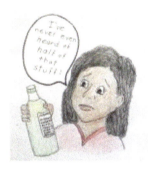

Roxy tries to read the label

- *"When I focused on eating real foods, my athletic performance soared."*[4]

- Start reading labels to find out what is in the foods you eat.

- Foods are best in their simplest form—whole fruits, veggies, and whole grains, for example. These can be called **real foods** or **whole foods.**

- **Whole foods** fuel your brain for **top mental focus** and positive attitude.

- Read labels and *especially avoid* HFCS (high fructose corn syrup), aspartame, trans fats, and ingredients you can't pronounce.

- Focus on foods that are "**nutrient dense**" (packed with vitamins) Examples: peanut butter on whole grain bread, sweet potatoes, black beans, brown rice, kale, eggs, sardines. If nutrient dense foods aren't on your usual menu, try a new recipe. (See chapter five.)

- Don't eat the same few foods every day. **Eat a variety** of high-quality foods to keep all your body systems in top form.

• How Do the World's Top Athletes Perform at their Best?

Coach and nutritionist Matt Fitzgerald interviewed many top athletes and learned they practice these **five habits**.[5] Join the ranks of these winners by following in their footsteps.

- They eat from all six food groups. (No fad diets allowed. They are not vegetarians.)

- They choose high quality foods. (You can benefit from this, too.)

- They eat a carb-centered diet. You might already do this, but are they *high quality* carbs?

- They eat enough to fuel their exercise needs. If you are trying to lose weight, cut back on low quality foods first. But when your body needs energy, choose wisely among the high quality carbohydrates.

- They tailor their diet to meet their individual needs. Food allergies obviously should be considered. Trying to lose excess weight or to gain more weight will affect your choices.

EAT TO STAY WELL

> EATING WELL IS THE KEY TO A LIFETIME OF GOOD
> HEALTH.

Don't let a cold or flu keep you on the bench! How can you stay well?

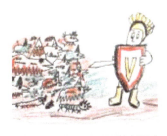

Here they come, all those
germs!

You have a complicated **immune system** lurking in your gut. Picture this; your **good bacteria** battle all the **bad bacteria** that come along. Which side will win?

Feed your good bacteria with yogurt and fermented foods. If you've been on antibiotics for an infection, you killed all those good bacteria along with the bad ones. Replace them with probiotic capsules, yogurt, or fermented foods.

Avoid sugar, which feeds the bad bacteria, undermining your immune system.

HINT–if you feel a cold coming on, take extra vitamin C, vitamin D, and zinc.

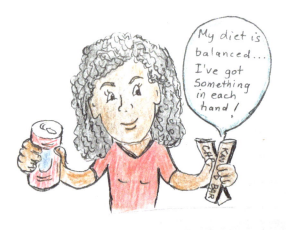

Roxy thinks her diet is balanced.What do you think?

WHY SHOULD I CHOOSE TO EAT REAL FOOD?

- The **immediate benefit** is better performance as an athlete.

- Any **overweight problems** are minimized without dieting.

- The **long-term health benefits** are many. Eating real food helps you avoid the "diseases of civilization". (For example, tooth decay, hypertension, fatty liver disease, diabetes, alzheimers, heart disease, and cancer. Yikes!)

- Eat **real food** most of the time so you can treat yourself on special occasions.

Beware of these health-robbers

- **soft drinks**, because they supply calories but have zero nutrition

- **aspartame**, because it has bad side effects

- **cookies, cake, pie**, all are high in refined carbs, low in fiber, vitamins, minerals
- **candy** has lots of carbs but zero nutrition
- **doughnuts** have refined carbs (no fiber, few vitamins), and unhealthy fat
- most **breakfast cereals** have a high sugar content and are low in fiber
- most **energy bars** have a high sugar content (gives a sugar high followed by fatigue)
- **sugar** in its many forms, (HFCS, sucrose, dextrose, etc.) promotes heart disease and diabetes, and it undermines the immune system
- **fried foods** and **chips** have unhealthful fat
- **processed meat** (this includes ham, cold cuts, bacon, chicken nuggets, hot dogs, lunchmeat) all have unhealthful additives

  - Beware=**be aware** that things on the list are not the best fuel for your growing body. Can you ever eat them? Yes, as a treat. These foods are tasty and available so eating whole foods is harder–**but you can do it**!

HOW CAN I CHANGE BAD EATING HABITS?

* Keep a food journal for three days to see what and when (and maybe why) you eat. Don't forget to count snacks.

- **Decide** which things to change.
- **Write down** one bad food you often consume and substitute something better in its place.

- **Ask a partner** to help—by keeping you honest or joining your "fitness club".

- **Be prepared** with a healthful snack when the hunger pangs strike and you're sure you will starve.

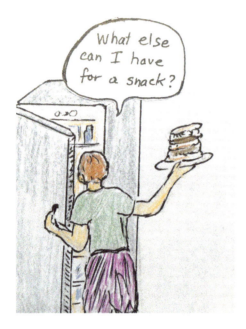

Rocky is having a growth spurt. Will he choose
a healthful snack?

Suggestions— Nuts, apple, banana, whole-grain crackers, raisins, popcorn, cheese sticks, veggies and dip.

- **Challenge a teammate** to see who can improve food choices the most.

- **Request** the "chief cook" at your house to help you change bad habits.

- **Volunteer** to prepare a healthful recipe to share with the family.

- Be willing to **try something new**! How hard can that be? Easier than push-ups!

- New habits take 21-30 days to establish, so **don't give up!**

TAKE THE PLEDGE

- **Remember, you have a million-dollar body. If you take care of it *now* it will last a long time.**

I WILL START TODAY TO....

Change this bad eating habit.

_____

Learn to like this healthful food and start eating it often.

– _____

Make food choices on the basis of what's good for me.

Date_____Signed_____

***ChooseMyPlate.gov* lets you and your friends create a club and track your progress.**

- [1] Fitzgerald, *The Endurance Diet,* p. 100

- [2] Ryan, *Sports Nutrition for Endurance Athletes,* p. 119.

- [3] Clark, *Sports Nutrition Guidebook,* p. 143.

- [4] Weiler and Mardigan, *Real Fit Kitchen,* p. 36.

- [5] Fitzgerald, *The Endurance Diet,* pp. 145-152.

3. Training Your Body

TRAINING

Training is the second way to improve your **endurance and energy.** The well-trained body is ready for action. Effective training includes these **three steps.**

*****Warm-up** for ten to fifteen minutes to get the blood pumping to your muscles.

*****Stretch** all the muscles you will use in your sport to keep them flexible. Stretching before exercise helps prevent injuries, too.

*****Cool down** after heavy exercise by walking or doing light exercise. This step prevents blood pooling in the legs. Rest between exercise sessions to allow refueling and repair of muscles.

How to Stretch

- Each time you exercise, tiny injuries happen in muscles. When these heal, the muscle is a tiny bit shorter. Stretch them out again. Here's how;

- Choose which muscles to stretch according to your sport's needs.

- Stretch the muscles you'll be using.

- Allow for fifteen minutes of stretching before exercise.

- Do the stretch slowly, not bouncing, and never to the point of pain.

- Hold the stretch for 20-60 seconds.

- Do not stretch very sore or injured muscles.

FLEXIBILITY EXERCISES

*Muscle–stretching exercises (see box above) will keep your *muscles* flexible.

*Range-of-motion exercises keep your *joints* flexible.

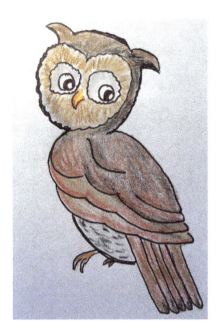

Can you turn your head around as far as
an owl?

Try these for starters.

- Like an owl, turn your head far to the right, hold for ten seconds, then turn your head far to the left for ten seconds.

- Make your arms wind up like an airplane propeller.

- Turn the top half of your body as far to the left, then as far to the right, as you can go without pain. Hold for ten seconds and repeat five times.

- Stretch your right leg out, holding it a few inches from the floor. Point your toes and rotate your foot at the ankle, 5–10 times. Repeat with left foot.

- Reach your right arm across your chest around to your left shoulder blade. Hold for ten seconds. Reach your left arm around to your right shoulder blade. Hold for ten seconds.

•

Breathe better...Run faster

- **Stand up straight**. Keep your shoulders back. You will expand the space for your lungs and thus can breathe more efficiently.

- **Breathe deeply**. Many sports are "aerobic", meaning they keep your heart pumping steadily and demand oxygen.

- **Oxygen** is used by your cells to change your food into **usable energy**.

PLAYING A SPORT MAKES EXERCISE FUN!

Try several different sports to see where your skills fit best. You might choose a team sport or an individual sport.

*Track events   *Cross-country running   *High jump   *Broad jump   *Basketball
  *Football   *Baseball   *Soccer
                    *Bicycling   *LaCross
                    *Rowing   *Rugby
  *Golf   *Wrestling   *Cheerleading
        *Horseback riding   *Swimming
  *Surfing   *Rollerblading
*Hiking   *Skiing   *Rock climbing
          *Dancing   *Snowboarding   *Tennis
              *Martial arts   *Gymnastics
  *Weight lifting   *Ice skating   *Ice hockey   *Archery   *Diving
          *Shot put

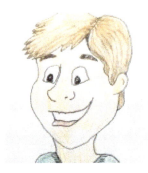

Rocky likes basketball

Which one is *your* favorite?

Rocky says...

- I like playing basketball, 'cause it keeps me in shape.
- My teammates point out skills I need to work on, and coach helps me learn them.
- Our team might make it to the state level this year, since we're playing well together.
- Coach tells me to keep up the good work!

HEART MUSCLE TRAINING

*Exercise until you are breathing hard.

*Continue exercising at that rate for thirty minutes.

*Train this way three times a week.

STRENGTH TRAINING

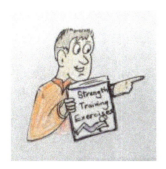

Coaches have good ideas

*Strength training exercises** improve your body's ability to perform.

Method—*overload* the muscle you are training, making your body carry extra weight during your training sessions. This increases **three things**: 1. Muscular **endurance** 2. Muscle **power** 3. muscle **strength**

*The best training exercises will mimic the sport you are training for. Examples–runners can add leg weights, basketball players can use arm weights, soccer players can kick a heavier ball. Plan your own exercises tailored to your sport.

*Strengthen the muscles you will use. Try these exercises for all-around training.

*Push–ups	*Step–ups
*Pull–ups	*Lunges
*Sit–ups	*Squats
*Resistance exercises	

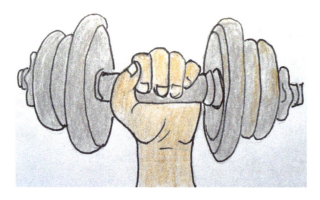

Lifting dumbbells gives muscles a workout

*There is **a right way** and **many wrong ways** to do each exercise. Ask your coach or look online for help.

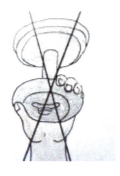

The wrong way!

RESISTANCE TRAINING

Resistance exercises are those which move your muscles against opposition, like

* your own weight   *gravity   *dumbbells
*elastic bands

***Resistance training** helps athletes gain muscle mass. A side benefit is an increase in strength.

*Simple resistance exercises include push-ups, jumping jacks, and lifting dumbbells or gallon jugs of water.

Learning a New Skill

- Learning a new skill is a hard task.

- Seek out a good coach so you can learn it right the first time.

- Hunt books on the skill written by professionals who can give inside tips.

- Practice, practice, practice.

- Don't get discouraged when the skill is harder than you expected.

- Practice the new skill along with your other routines, so you don't lose your old skills.

- Sleep well after the skill-learning sessions; your brain will retain what you have learned.

- When you've learned the basics, see if you can teach another; teachers always learn more than their pupils.

SKILL DEVELOPMENT EXERCISES

Skills include   *Coordination
*Agility
  *Balance   *Visual Tracking.   *Foot speed

You already have these skills, but to *improve* them, try these exercises.

- Jump rope. Mix it up by hopping, skipping, and going extra-fast.

- Run through an obstacle course you set up. Increase your speed.

- Dribble a soccer ball through the obstacle course.

- Dribble a basketball through an obstacle course on the court.

- "Flamingo stand" on one leg, with the opposite foot braced against the thigh. See if you can balance for ten seconds. Try to rotate your body by sliding the standing foot in a circle.

- Softball throw. Make a large target, stand back 15 feet or so, throw the ball as hard as you can and still hit the target. Now back up and try again.

> ### Roxy says
>
>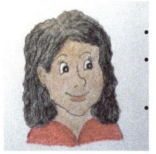
> Here's why I play soccer :
>
> - I want to get some exercise.
>
> - My best friend is on the team and that makes it fun.
>
> - The coach knows how to get the best performance out of me.
>
> - I hope to get a scholarship, since that would really help me pay my way through college.

MENTAL FITNESS

You've seen it—one team is **up** and ready for action. They exude confidence.

The other team is sluggish, they let little things annoy them, and they make stupid mistakes and mental errors.

What's the difference? *Attitude.* <mark>Attitude is key in any sport.</mark>

Negative attitude does three things, all bad.

*Negative attitude **saps energy.**

*Negative attitude **hurts team play.**

*Negative attitude **causes mistakes in judgment.**

TRAINING FOR POSITIVE MENTAL ATTITUDE

How can you have a **positive mental attitude**, even when things are not going well?

Give yourself a pep talk with these positive facts:

*Look at the big picture.** Learn from the problem, but don't dwell on it too much.

*Find the humor** in the situation. (Be careful not to mock others, however.)

*Remind yourself that *how you play* is more important than whether you win.

*Competition** forces you to work harder toward your goal.

*Competition** reveals your skills, strengths, and weaknesses.

Remember, *winning* isn't beating everyone else, that's just coming in first. **Winning is when you keep going after a setback.**"[1]

Read an inspiring sports biography

- *The Boys in the Boat: Nine Americans and Their Epic Quest for Gold at the 1936 Olympics*, by Daniel Brown.

- *For the Glory: Eric Liddell's Journey from Olympic Champion to Modern Martyr*, by Duncan Hamilton.

- *Unbroken: An Olympian's Journey from Airman to Castaway, to Captive*, by Laura Hillenbrand.

OBSTACLES

Obstacles will *always* come on the way to your goal.

*Identify** physical obstacles, plan how to overcome them.

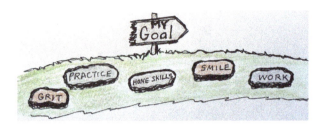

Steps toward your goal

*Identify mental obstacles, then remove them.

*Imagine the steps to your goal or your team's goal.

*Mentally prepare for the unexpected–don't let things throw you for a loop.

"Luxury and comfort are not goals, they're distractions.[2]

REDEFINE FAILURE...It may really be an opportunity

- Failure is a way to **learn your**

weaknesses so you can work to strengthen them.

- **Choose your reaction** to failure and use it to improve your game.

- Seek advice from coaches, teammates, and parents.

- **When opportunity knocks**, be ready to open the door; don't sit on the couch just because it is more comfortable.

TEAM PRACTICES

Be proactive as you participate in regular team practices. How?

*Ask the coach** to point out your weaknesses and how to overcome them.

*Practice each skill** as soon as you learn it, making sure you do it correctly.

*Practice ways you and the others can **work smoothly as a team.**

*Be the team cheerleader** and encourage your teammates.

DISCIPLINE is PRACTICING THE KNOWLEDGE YOU'VE LEARNED.

Have you heard this? "Sitting is the new smoking." In other words, it's bad to sit around.

Try these ideas to **integrate exercise** into your daily life *between* sports seasons.

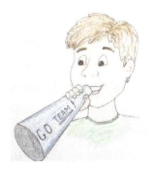

Rocky cheers you on

- Stretch your back muscles as you bend over to tie your shoes.

- When you brush your teeth, do range-of-motion exercises for your neck.

- Do range-of-motion exercises for your torso as you shower.

- Do leg lifts before you hop out of bed each morning.

- Walk briskly to wherever you are going.

- Do squats and jumping jacks while waiting in line for the bus.

- Rocky and Roxy say, "DON'T JUST SIT THERE, DO SOMETHING!"

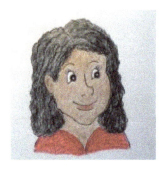

Keep active and stay fit

[1] Davis, *Raising Men*, p.166.

[2] Davis, *Raising Men*, p.182.

4. Special Conditions

Other factors to consider for overall fitness

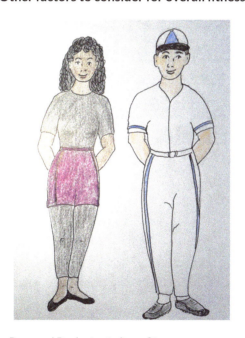

Roxy and Rocky try to keep fit

INJURY PREVENTION

Weak muscles are more injury-prone. Lack of fitness is

the reason many injuries happen at the beginning of the season, even during the first few practices.

Don't let an injury sideline you from a season of play.

Stretch and warm up before exercise

*Start warming up slowly and then increase the pace.

*Stretching fills muscles with blood, makes them pliable.

*Stretching heats up muscles to prepare them for work.

*Warming up cuts down on sprains and strains.

"A warm-up will improve speed, balance, agility, strength, and endurance."[1]

A Few Case Histories

Grant dribbled the basketball down the court, slowed by his extra pounds. Coach had to sub him out a few minutes later, since he was red-faced, winded, and complained of pain in his side and a bad leg cramp. Coach suggested doing warm-up exercises and cutting back on the sweets.

Lashawn sprinted ahead of the pack of runners. She kept up the pace for half the race, but began to slow down and lost the lead. Fatigue increased and her legs felt like lead weights. Several more runners passed her, but she could not run any faster. She was glad she didn't come in dead last. That energy bar had *not* helped, as the ad promised.

Trent raced out to the field for the first practice of the year. He wanted to show the coach he was ready for a starting position. But after a few minutes, he felt his ankle twist painfully as he fell. With help, he limped off the field. Coach iced the injury and reminded him it's best to warm up before running hard.

IMMEDIATE TREATMENT FOR INJURIES

*USE THE **R-I-C-E** STRATEGY (**R**est, **I**ce, **C**ompress, and **E**levate)*

*<u>Rest</u> the injured body part.

*<u>Ice</u> the area, first protecting it with a towel.

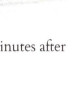

*<u>Compress</u> the injury with an elastic bandage around the ice. This limits swelling.   Remove for fifteen minutes after the first half hour. Repeat for up to three hours.

*<u>Elevate</u> the injury to help drain excess fluid.

DURING RECOVERY FROM AN INJURY

* Adjust caloric intake down if you are less active.

* Increase fruit and vegetable intake for faster injury recovery.

* Carbohydrates help with muscle repair, but beware of "empty" calories. (Your carbs should come from whole foods, not refined snacks.)

* Vitamin C is needed to produce collagen for cartilage, tendons, and bones.

* Vitamin C is needed to produce red blood cells.

* Zinc promotes healing of wounds.

AVOIDING CRAMPS

*Cramps may indicate you need more magnesium.

*You may have overstretched a muscle. Warm-up and pre-stretch next time.

*You may have lost too much salt through sweat. Try a salty snack.

* You may be dehydrated. Cold water will rehydrate you the fastest.

DEHYDRATION–DON'T LET IT HAPPEN TO YOU

Dehydration has many symptoms.

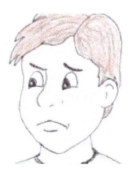

Rocky's grumpy–he might be dehydrated

*Cramps   *Sore muscles   *Confusion
  *Light-headedness or dizziness
  *Fatigue (also caused by low iron or poor nutrition)
  *Headache   *Dry mouth
  *Grumpiness *Sleepiness

Key Takeaways

- Even a small amount of dehydration affects your speed, energy, and performance.

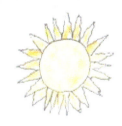

The hot sun saps energy

HOT WEATHER EXERCISE

*Avoid the midday sun if possible.

*Rest ten minutes every hour.

*Drink 8–10 oz. of water every 20 minutes.

*Use sunscreen.

*Wear light-weight, light-colored clothes.

*Be alert for nausea or light-headedness indicating heat stroke.

DANGER OF OVERTRAINING

Your body needs rest between periods of intense exercise. But what if you're in a tournament? Minimize the stress by getting extra sleep and eating extra high-quality carbs.

If you lose your appetite, can't sleep well, have mood swings, are fatigued, and often get sick, *you might be training too hard*.

CONCUSSIONS

STOP PLAYING AFTER A HEAD BUMP

Watch for these symptoms, which may show up immediately or later.

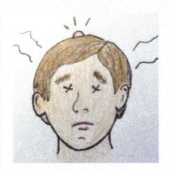

This player's head bump may mean a concussion

- headache

- dizziness

- lights and noise bother you

- vision blurry

- sick to your stomach

- can't concentrate or remember

- overly emotional reactions

- confused

- sleep problems

Report the symptoms to coach or parent

SELF-CONTROL

Every athlete exercises self-control in all things...I discipline my body and keep it under control.   I Corinthians 9:25,27.

Self-discipline is necessary to **TURN AWAY** from things that **undermine your health,** (either physical or mental.)

*DRUGS   *Junk Food   *Pornography *ALCOHOL   *Distracted Driving   *Bad attitude   *SMOKING *Cheating on Sleep   *The bad habit you need to stop

A MAN WITHOUT SELF-CONTROL IS LIKE A CITY BROKEN INTO AND LEFT WITHOUT WALLS.   Proverbs 25:28

GROWTH SPURTS

- Young athletes go through periods when their bodies grow faster than usual.

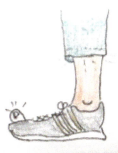

Two signs of a growth spurt here.

- Girls usually have a growth spurt around age 10 or 11.

- Boys usually have their growth spurts at age 12 or 13.

- YOU MAY BE HAVING A GROWTH SPURT IF.....

- Your feet are growing out of your shoes

- Your legs are too long for your pants

- Your arms are too long for your long-sleeved shirts

- You are always hungry

NUTRITION IS EVEN MORE IMPORTANT NOW

- **Your bones** are getting longer, they need calcium.

- **Your brain** is busier, it needs vitamins and minerals and good fats.

- **Your muscles** are thickening, so keep them strong by exercising and eating well.

- **You are gaining weight**. Make sure it is healthy weight by eating from the six food groups and avoiding empty calories.

- **Your skin** may develop acne, another reminder to eat high quality food.

SLEEP

- Athletes who got 10 hours of sleep ran faster, had less fatigue, and more stamina.[2]

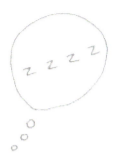

Sleep is important for good
health

DON'T CHEAT YOURSELF ON SLEEP

Both exercise and growth spurts put demands on your body for SLEEP.

*Plan ahead.** Get the homework done, the test studied for, and get **ten hours** of sleep each night.

*During sleep** your body **repairs** those little muscle injuries caused by exercise.

*During sleep your brain **reviews the skills** you learned, so you learn them better.

*Sleep deprivation** lowers performance in athletics and lowers concentration in school. It can be **dangerous** if you're driving a car.

*Beware of **blue-screen light** before bedtime, it tends to keep you awake.

*Don't depend on **caffeine** to wake you up the next morning or keep you awake during the day. Get adequate sleep instead.

*Listen** to your body when it says, "I'm sleepy."

FOOD CRAVINGS

Why can't you eat just one chip? Salty snacks make you want more. Sugary treats work in a similar way. **Conquer food cravings by eating real food.**

Food cravings are different from hunger pains. Cravings are when your body demands a certain thing and you are powerless to resist. Food cravings disappear when you choose your menu from **all six food groups.** Why? Because the cravings mean **something is missing** from your diet. Whole foods will provide all the nutrients your body needs.

TRYING TO LOSE WEIGHT

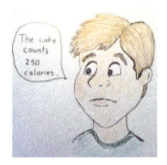

Will Rocky cut those cake calories?

Counting calories doesn't usually work.

You need a *whole new outlook on food.*

Ask yourself, "Why do I eat what I eat?"

*Because it tastes good?

*Because it is **real food** and promotes good health?

Learn to like what is good for you. Is that harder to do than those push-ups coach assigned?

Try These Ideas

Proven Strategies to Help You Lose Weight

1. Drink a **glass of water** before your meal.
2. Use a **smaller plate** and fill it only once, (with no piling.)
3. Eat **s l o w l y**, taking small bites and chewing well. Eating is not a race!
4. **Stop eating** when you're full, even if it still tastes like "more."
5. **Try this exercise** right after you finish that first small plateful. ***Push back*** from the table, get up and start helping with the dishes. (Your mom will love you for that!)
6. After a meal, **don't sit**. Instead, do some light exercise.
7. Sugar is what makes us fat, so **cut back** drastically on all the sweets.
8. **Take this challenge**: Instead of a BIG piece of dessert, take an **inch square** serving. Use a teeny spoon to eat it. Savor each tiny bite! Doesn't your tiny bit taste just as good as a huge chunk?
9. **Don't starve yourself** to try to get thin–eat a balanced diet of healthy foods, to fuel your body for growth and the demands of exercise.
10. Choose foods that fill you up but are still healthful. Many on the **superfoods** list fit this category.
11. **Get a partner** to share your triumphs. (Or write in your food journal).
12. Avoid **mindless eating**; watching TV or movie with low-quality snacks.

SNACKS BEFORE A GAME

- It is important to keep up energy, before and during exercise.

- Pregame/pre-exercise; choose high quality carbs which digest quickly, readily available for muscle energy.

- Choose low-fat foods, since fat slows digestion. Don't forget to hydrate, too.

- Plan ahead for snacks; **carry-alongs**; *banana *apple *orange *whole-grain crackers *peanut butter on whole-grain bread *100% fruit juice *popcorn *yogurt (w/o sugar)

CHALLENGE

KEEP A FOOD JOURNAL AND SCORE YOURSELF

Write down your breakfast, lunch, dinner, and snacks each day.

- Give yourself a **plus one** for every serving of Super Foods (see chapter 5)

- Give yourself **plus two** for each day you had something from each of the six food groups.

- Give yourself a **plus one** every time you try a new healthful food.

- Give yourself a **minus two** every time you gobble a serving of Low Quality food.

Can you increase your daily score as you improve your eating habits?

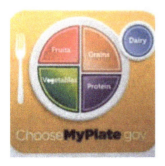

This government website has great ideas for you

Try online food tracking–use SuperTracker on the website, **choosemyplate.gov**

[1] Southmayd, *Sports Health, The Complete Book of Athletic Injuries,* p. 56.

[2] De Sena, Joe. *Spartan Fit! 30 Days,* p.94.

5. Super Foods and Recipes

Look at the A to Z Super Foods list below. Choose which food group they belong in.

*Meats/fish *Dairy *Nuts, seeds, oils *Fruits *Vegetables *Whole Grains

SUPER FOODS FROM A to Z

Super Foods are packed with nutrients.

How many of these A to Z Super Foods are on the menu at your house?

A is for Avocado. This fruit has healthy fat, potassium, and fiber.

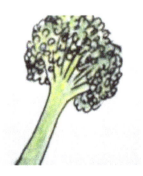

Broccoli gets a 5 star rating

B is for Broccoli. It has twice the vitamin C found in an orange and almost as much calcium as whole milk.

B is also for Beans. Beans are high in protein, fiber, B-vitamins, and antioxidants.

C is for Chia seeds These tiny seeds are high in omega-3 oil and antioxidants.

C is also for Coconut oil This oil is a healthy fat, good for energy and brain work.

D is for Dandelion Greens Yes, this common weed has amazing amounts of vitamin K, and lots of other good things, too.

E is for Eggs Eggs have protein, healthy fat, and B vitamins.

F is for Fermented foods Sauerkraut and other fermented foods aid digestion, boost immune system.

G is for Garlic. Garlic helps the immune system and acts as a natural antibiotic.

H is for Honey Honey is an energy booster (use sparingly).

I is for Iced smoothies Blenderize your fruits and veggies and add other health boosters.

J is for Juices (with no extra sugar.) Fruit juices are a portable carb source, especially good for athletes.

K is for Kiwi This fruit is packed with vitamins, A, C, E, and K.

K is also for Kale Kale is high in vitamin K, vitamin C, and fiber.

L is for Lentils. This nutrient-dense food has protein, fiber, and iron.

M is for Milk This and other dairy products are a good source of calcium.

N is for Nibs of cacao (raw chocolate source) This has twenty times more antioxidant power than blueberries.

O is for Oats Oats have complex carbohydrates and fiber.

P is for Pineapple Fresh pineapple is a great source of vitamin C and other nutrients.

Q is for Quinoa This seed has all nine amino acids, plus iron, manganese, and B-12.

R is for Real foods Add real foods from all 6 groups to your menu.

S is for Strawberries Berries have fiber, antioxidants, and vitamins.

S is also for Salmon and Sardines These fish have healthy fat, which is good for energy and brain work.

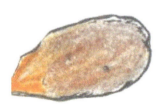

S is also for Sweet Potatoes. This food is a super source of vitamin A. They also have vitamin C, D, calcium, and magnesium.

T is for Tomatoes This delicious fruit has lots of vitamins C, A, and K, plus other micronutrients.

U is for Ugli fruit This and other citrus-family fruits have lots of vitamin C plus calcium and vitamin A.

V is for Vegetables. Veggies come in many varieties, colors, and shapes. Try a new one; it is sure to be vitamin-packed.

W is for Walnuts Walnuts and other nuts, (raw), have antioxidants, B vitamins, folic acid, and fiber.

W is also for Whole grain foods Whole grain foods are already rich in vitamins, so don't have to be "enriched" with extra vitamins.

X is for a mystery food See what you discover as you try new things.

Y is for Yogurt Yogurt has calcium, B vitamins, probiotics, and zinc. Choose unsweetened and add fruit.

Z is for Zucchini This veggie is a great source of B-vitamins and has more potassium than a banana.

TRY A NEW RECIPE

Smoothies, Shakes, and Frozen Treats

Use a blender or food processor to whip up a new favorite–a **health shake**. Try one for a power-packed breakfast.

Create your own recipes using these guidelines:

1/2 to 1 Cup *liquid* (Water, milk, juice, or nut milk)

1/2 to 3/4 Cup *fruit,* chopped (Pineapple, lemon, banana, berries, etc.) Tart and sweet fruits combine well.

1/4 to 3/4 Cup *veggies*, chopped (kale, cucumber, beet, dandelion greens, kraut)

Sneak in small amounts of these as desired: chia seeds, oatmeal, yogurt.

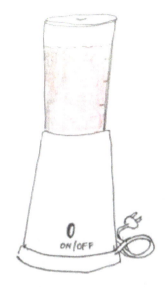

Place all ingredients in blender, *blend* until well-mixed. Drink right away.

Make a big batch and freeze extra in ice-cube trays for delicious freezer pops.

Creative Salad Ideas

- **Salads** are a great way to eat lots of veggies. Forget those boring salads of iceberg lettuce and pale tomatoes! Choose from the veggie list below, add a few extras to make it unique, and add protein to make it a meal.

- **VEGGIES**

- tomatoes cut into bite-sized pieces

- cucumber slices

- carrots, sliced thin

- green onions, chopped

- celery, 1/2" slices

- kale, chopped fine

- broccoli or cauliflower, bite-sized florets

- lettuce and mixed greens, torn into pieces

Roxy whips up a salad

- **PROTEIN**

- Cooked chicken, pork, or beef shreds

- Kidney, red, or black beans

- cheese, shredded or sliced

- hard-boiled eggs, sliced

- nuts, raw

- cooked quinoa
- **SURPRISE EXTRAS**

• grapes or raisins	*strawberries	*raspberries
• pineapple	*pickled beets	*mint leaves
• sauerkraut	*tart cherries	*sunflower seeds
• zucchini, yellow squash		

Make-your-own Salad Dressing

- **Basic salad dressing** Make your own dressings so you can avoid unhealthy ingredients. Mix the oil and vinegar for a base, then add a *small selection* of the other ingredients, tasting as you go, to create your own salad dressing.

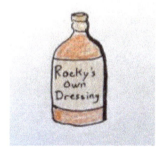

Help Rocky name his dressing

- olive oil, 2/3 cup
- apple cider vinegar, 1/3 cup
- salt and pepper
- honey, 1 Tablespoon

- Greek yogurt, a lot or a little

- mustard or ketchup to taste

- hot sauce for spiciness

- pickle relish

- chia seeds

- sour cream

- grated ginger root makes an extra zing

- chopped garlic

- spices, such as cumin, chili powder, garlic powder, or curry powder

Bread, Pizza, and Pretzels

- Bread made from whole grains is a healthful and delicious source of carbohydrates. With a few simple ingredients you can make some mouth-watering goodies. Even if you don't have a bread machine, you will be able to bake the following recipes. If you do have a bread machine, follow directions for making basic dough, baking it in your oven, not the machine.

BASIC DOUGH

In a large bowl, pour

1 1/2 cups lukewarm (90 degrees) water

Add 1 teaspoon vinegar

Add 2 teaspoons sugar

Sprinkle 2 teaspoons of dry yeast on the water

Wait 5 minutes, till the yeast bubbles.

Add 2 tablespoons olive oil or liquid shortening

Optional; 1 tablespoon of gluten makes the bread rise higher.

Add 4 cups white whole wheat flour* (more or less, depending on the dough) (We recommend *King Arthur* brand.)

Add 1 teaspoon salt

Stir the ingredients together. Form them into a ball. Add more water or flour as needed until the dough is soft but not sticky.

Knead the dough. You can use it as exercise if you do it right! That means push it down *hard* with the heels of your hands, fold it in half, and do it again until the bread is smooth and elastic. This may take **5-10 minutes.**

Return dough to an oiled bowl, turn once to oil the dough, cover with a damp towel and put in a warm (90 degrees) place. During this rise cycle (maybe **40-45 minutes** or until the dough has doubled in size,) you can decide what to make with the dough.

SANDWICH ROLLS

Divide dough into 14 or so pieces. Tuck the outside edges under each roll to make the top smooth, then flatten. Place on greased cookie sheets, allow to rise again till doubled in size. **Bake at 375 degrees 24-26 minutes**, until lightly browned. Cool thoroughly before storing in container. This bread has no preservatives (that's one reason it's so yummy), so if you have any left after 4 days, refrigerate to prevent mold.

PIZZA DOUGH

Grease two cookie sheets. Divide dough in half. Gently stretch each piece into a circle, flattening and stretching as you go. Let it rest a while if it is too stretchy. When you have it as large as you want it, pinch an edge all around. Add a layer of pizza sauce, cheese, and toppings, like onions, green peppers, hot peppers, pepperoni, cooked sausage. **Bake 15-20 minutes at 375 degrees** until lightly browned. Cool 5 minutes before cutting.

SOFT PRETZELS

Divide dough into 16 pieces.

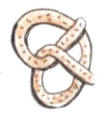

Yummy soft pretzels are a favorite

Roll each piece into a 14″ rope. Loop the rope around and cross it at the bottom to make a pretzel. Place each on a parchment paper-lined sheet. Allow to rise till double. Then carefully place each one in **boiling water for a minute** (this makes them chewy). Place on baking sheet, brush with egg wash (1 beaten egg, 1 tablespoon water) , sprinkle with coarse salt, and bake for **12-15 minutes, at 450 degrees.**

*Other options to add variety.

Add 3 tablespoons sunflower seeds to the roll dough

Add 2 tablespoons chia seed to the roll dough

Add 1 tablespoon oregano to the pizza dough

Add 3 tablespoons grated parmesan cheese to the soft pretzel dough

Gourmet Roasted Vegetables

Transform any vegetable into a gourmet dish by roasting it with oil and herbs.

*Garlic

Peel, brush with oil, bake at **350 degrees for 10 minutes**.

*Sweet potato

Scrub, do not peel potato, cut into 1″ chunks. In bowl, melt 1.5 tablespoons coconut oil, add two teaspoons cinnamon, 2 teaspoons salt, 1 teaspoon chia seed. Stir chunks in until coated. Spread evenly on baking sheet. **Bake at 350 degrees for 40 minutes**, turning once.

*Brussels sprouts

Brush with oil, bake at **375 degrees for 12 minutes,** or until tender.

*Butternut squash

Peel and cut into 1″ chunks, brush with melted butter, **bake at 375 degrees for 15-20 minutes** until tender.

*Roasted white potato and onion

Preheat oven to **475 degrees**.

In a bowl, combine 1 tablespoon chopped fresh thyme, 2 tablespoons chopped fresh rosemary, 4 tablespoons olive oil, and 2 tablespoons apple cider vinegar (or balsamic vinegar).

Scrub potato, cut into 1″ chunks. Quarter the onion, separate into pieces. Stir vegetables into the oil and spice mixture to coat. Spread evenly in roasting pan. Sprinkle with salt and pepper. **Bake 35-40 minutes, stirring every 10 minutes**, until potatoes are browned.

Energy Bars

- Have you read the label on those expensive energy bars? They may contain all kinds of things you don't want to eat. It's healthier and cheaper to make your own.

• *Peanut butter energy bars (no bake)

1/2 cup natural peanut butter	1/2 cup mashed berries	1/4 cup chia seeds
	2 tablespoons honey	1/2 cup rolled oats
1/4 cup dried cranberries		1/4 cup peanuts, chopped

Mash the berries, add the chia seeds, allow to set 15 minutes. Mix all ingredients. Pat flat onto cookie sheet. Refrigerate 30 minutes before cutting. Store in fridge or freezer.

- ### *Almond energy bars (no bake)

- 1 cup pitted dates

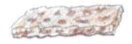

Energy bars are portable

- 1/4 cup honey

- 1/4 cup creamy peanut butter

- 1 cup coarsely chopped roasted almonds

- 1 1/2 cups rolled oats (Toast in oven for 10 minutes if you like.)

- 1 tablespoon water

- Blend dates in food processor until chopped. Mix peanut butter, honey, and water, pour over oats in a bowl. Add dates, breaking them apart to mix. Line an 8″ x 8″ pan with waxed paper or plastic wrap. Put mixture in pan, press down hard to flatten the mix and bond it. Refrigerate for 20 minutes before cutting into bars. Makes 8 bars.

*Nutty fruit bars (no bake)

- 1 cup pitted dates

- 1 cup toasted (or raw) walnuts

- 1 cup dried cranberries

- 1 cup unsweetened coconut shreds

Process all ingredients until well-chopped. Add 1 tablespoon of water and process again a minute or so until mixture will hold together when pressed with fingers. Place mix in plastic lined pan, press hard to form it into bars. Refrigerate an hour before cutting. Makes 16 bars.

*Oatmeal energy bars (baked)

- 1 cup whole wheat flour

- 1/4 cup oats

- 1 teaspoon baking powder

- 1 egg, beaten

- 1/4 cup (4 tablespoons) honey

- 1/3 cup nut butter

- 1 teaspoon vanilla extract

- 2 tablespoons melted butter

- 2 tablespoons milk

- 1/4 cup dried fruit (like raisins)

- 1/4 cup chopped walnuts

- 1/4 cup sunflower or pumpkin seeds

Mix the dry ingredients in a small bowl. Mix the egg, honey, nut butter, vanilla, melted butter, and milk in a large bowl, very well, until smooth. Stir in the fruit and seeds and nuts. Press the mixture into an 8 inch by 8 inch greased pan.

Bake at 350 degrees for 25 minutes, testing to see whether a toothpick comes out clean. If it doesn't, bake a little longer. Cut into eight bars. Take along for after school, before practice, and watch your energy zoom!

Wraps, Pita Pockets, and Tortillas

TACOS

- 8 whole wheat tortillas, 7" size
- *1 lb. hamburger, browned and broken apart
- *1 tablespoon taco seasoning, with 3 tablespoons of water
- In separate bowls: *chopped kale and chopped lettuce
-                                    *shredded cheese
-                                    *cherry tomatoes, halved
-                                    *Greek yogurt with finely chopped chives
-                                    *Salsa

Serve the seasoned meat and the other ingredients in bowls. Put some of everything in the tortilla , but be careful not to fill it too full! Wrap tightly, folding under the bottom. Enjoy!

TUNA WRAP

- One 7 oz. can of tuna
- Add 4 tablespoons Greek yogurt
- Stir in 1/3 cup chopped sauerkraut, drained
- Add 1/2 cup finely chopped celery
- Add 1 or 2 hardboiled eggs, chopped
- Add a squirt of hot pepper sauce (optional)
- Add 2 tablespoons pickle relish (optional)
- Stuff into pita pockets or roll into whole grain wraps. Yum!
- OR, serve in the middle of a tomato "flower".
- You won't even be able to taste the "weird" ingredients, but the kraut and yogurt will stoke your beneficial bacteria!

Super Side Dishes

COWBOY CAVIAR–a colorful salad with a southwest flair.

Mix the oil, vinegar, honey, and spices in a large bowl. Add the vegetables. Mix well. Add the chopped cilantro. Refrigerate at least an hour to let the flavors blend.

- 6 tablespoons olive oil
- 3 tablespoons apple cider vinegar

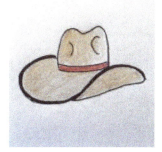

Cowboys like this salad

- 2 tablespoons honey
- 1 teaspoon chili powder
- 1 teaspoon salt
- 3/4 cup corn (drained if canned)
- 1 cup chopped sweet pepper, any color
- 1 red onion, diced
- 1 pound roma tomatoes, diced
- 1 (15 oz.) can red beans, drained
- 1 (15 oz) can black beans, drained
- * 1 cup chopped cilantro–stir in right before serving

BROCCOLI and APPLE SALAD

This simple salad is fast and easy to make and tastes good, too, of course!

- 1 cup broccoli, cut into small florets
- 1 cup tart apple, cut into small pieces
- 1/4 cup Greek yogurt
- 2 teaspoons apple cider vinegar
- 2 teaspoons honey
- 1/4 cup raisins
- 2 tablespoons walnuts, coarsely chopped.
- Stir all ingredients together and serve.

Main Dishes

KOREAN BULGOGI (FIRE STEAK)

- 1 lb. boneless chuck roast, sliced 1/4″ thick, (freeze 30 min. for easy slicing)
- Marinate for a few hours in 2 teaspoons olive oil, 2 tablespoons soy sauce, 1 teaspoon ginger (powdered or fresh-grated)
- Add thinly-sliced onions and thinly-sliced green pepper (a lot or a little)
- Fry in skillet, one layer at a time.
- Use the browned meat juice/ marinade to flavor the brown rice.
- Serve over brown rice.

TAOS SALMON CORNCAKES

- 1/2 cup cornmeal, microwaved for 30-45 seconds with 3/4 cup water, till thick
- In bowl, 1 (6 ounce) can of salmon, juice and all. Add;
- 1 tablespoon chopped onion.
- 2 tablespoons finely chopped green pepper
- 3 tablespoons finely chopped celery
- 2 eggs
- 2 teaspoons (more if you like) taco seasoning
- 1 teaspoon hot sauce.
- Mix well. Fry 3" patties of mixture on greased griddle, turning once.
- Just before serving, add slices of cojack cheese to the top.
- Warm salsa to serve over each corncake.

6. Look Ahead to the Future

Some day you will be grown up.

But **today** you are making decisions which affect your future.

You are becoming *what you will be* by the choices you make *starting today*.

Now is an important time in your life. Now is the time to think about the lessons you're learning.

ROXY SHARES THE LESSONS SHE'S LEARNED

- My body needs the right fuel to work properly, so I stay away from junk food. I've learned to like five new foods!

- I learned how to cook and I like it! Now I give my mom a break by fixing a healthy dinner several times a month.

- My grandma has diabetes and is on dialysis. Sugar is poison for her, and probably for me, too.

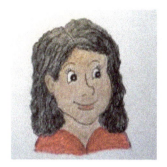

Roxy shares what she's learned

- I plan exercise into my daily routine to help my muscles to stay strong.

- Friends helped me through the rough places on my path,
                    so I want to help them. Now I have good ideas to share.

- I encourage others (and myself) to keep moving toward our goals.

- I *almost enjoy* doing the hard exercise things, since they help me toward my goal, a sports scholarship for college.

ROCKY SAYS HE'S MORE FIT TODAY

- I got rid of most of the flabby extra weight I had been carrying around.

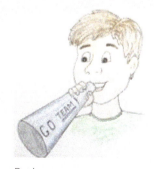

Rocky says...

- My coach talked to me about self-control in what I eat, so that helps me stay fit.

- I convinced my family to have a good breakfast with me every day.

- I learned more about nutrition and am more careful of what I eat.

- I surprised my mom by making energy bars for game day. Twice!

- My uncle has heart disease and it may run in the family, so I'm extra-careful about exercising and eating right.

- Everyone on our team needs to stay fit so we encourage each other.

- Between sport seasons, my buddy and I go mountain biking on a course nearby.

- How about you?

This book talks about how to **feed and exercise** our bodies. This helps *slow down* the march of time. But eventually our bodies will wear out.

But there is a part of us which will **last** *forever*. It would be useless to have a strong body but ignore our soul.

Jesus, the Bread of Life, promises to satisfy our soul-hunger.

> **Jesus said to them, "I am the bread of life; whoever comes to me shall not hunger, and whoever believes in me shall not thirst.   John 6:35**

THE PROBLEM–We live in a sinful world

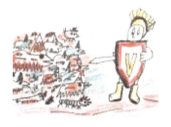

We see it even on the **microscopic level.** The **bad germs** attack, the **defenders** fight back.

We see it on the **worldwide level** in wars and acts of mass terrorism.

We see it on a **personal level** when we lose our temper or envy another's popularity.

Each person has a sinful heart because we are descended from Adam and Eve.

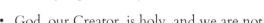

- Adam and Eve disobeyed God in the Garden of Eden. (We would have, too.)

- Each person who sins (every single human), is *already* condemned, even before Judgment Day.

- God, our Creator, is holy, and we are not.

For all have sinned and fall short of the glory of God.   Romans 3:23

THE SOLUTION

God's **perfect solution** to this **sin problem** was to send his **perfect, sinless Son** into the world.

> **John 14:6**
>
> Jesus said to him, I am the way, and the truth, and the life. No one comes to the Father except through me.

We can **trust Jesus Christ** to do what we cannot do. We can't earn God's forgiveness even by the very best of our good works.

We deserve death.

> **But God showed his love for us in that while we were still**
>
> **sinners, Christ died for us.   Romans 5:8**

MY RESPONSE

You needed to *take action* to get your physical body in top shape. But we can't do anything to change our sinful soul.

Instead, humbly claim the perfect righteousness of Jesus by believing he died for you.

> For God so loved the world that he gave his only Son, that whoever believes in him should not perish but have eternal life.   John 3:16

YOUR JOURNEY

If you have believed that Jesus took the punishment you deserved by dying in your place, then you are now a baby believer.

- **Baby believers grow by practicing skills, just like in sports**

- by **reading** God's love letter to you, **the Bible**.

- by **talking to God, your Heavenly Father** and to **Jesus** who sits at his right hand. He loves to hear from his children as they pray about everyday needs.

- by **fellowshipping** with other believers in a **church family**.

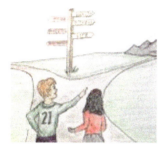

Begin by taking "baby steps" and soon you will grow as a Christian.

Rocky and Roxy make important life choices.

My Prayer

Dear God, Thank you for sending your Son, Jesus, to die in my place. Give me wisdom to take care of the amazing body you have given me so I can serve you. Amen.

Bibliography and Author's note

Bernardot, Dan, M.D. *Advanced Sports Nutrition.* Champaign, Illinois, Human Kinetics, 2006.

Clark, Nancy, MS, RD. *Sports Nutrition Guidebook, Fifth Edition.* Champaign, Illinois, Human Kinetics, 2014.

Davis, Eric. *Raising Men, Lessons Navy Seals Learned from Their Training and Taught to Their Sons.* New York, St. Martin's Press, 2016.

De Sena, Joe. *Spartan Fit! 30 Days. Transform Your Mind, Transform Your Body, Commit to Grit.* Boston, New York, Houghton Mifflin, 2016.

Fitzgerald, Matt. *The Endurance Diet, Discover the 5 Core Habits of the World's Greatest Athletes to Look, Feel, and Perform Better.* Boston, DaCapo Press, 2016.

Hagerman, Patrick. *Strength Training for Triathletes.* Boulder, Colorado, Velopress, 2015.

Lauren, Mark. *Body Fuel, Calorie-cycle Your Way to Reduced Body Fat and Greater Muscle Definition.* New York, Ballantine Books, 2016.

Rau, Dana Meachen. *Sports Nutrition for Teen Athletes, Eat Right to Take Your Game to the Next Level.* Mankato, Minnesota, Capstone Press, 2012.

Schwarzenegger, Arnold. *Arnold's Fitness for Kids Ages 11-14. A Guide to Health, Exercise, and Nutrition.* New York, Doubleday, 1993.

Southmayd, Wm, M.D. *Sports Health, the Complete Book of Athletic Injuries.* New York, Quick Fox, 1981.

★★★

Visit the author's website <ohiofrontierhistorylady.com>

Karen Meyer has written six other books for young readers. Discover the exciting stories of frontier history in *Conflict at Chillicothe, Battle at Blue Licks, Missing at Marietta,* and *Whispers at Marietta.* Explore the Underground Railroad in Ohio in *North to Freedom.* Meet Orville and Wilbur Wright in *The Tiara Mystery.*

The author enjoys hearing from readers! Leave comments on the website. <ohiofrontierhistorylady.com>

CPSIA information can be obtained
at www.ICGtesting.com
Printed in the USA
LVHW081039020119
602254LV00010B/346/P

9 780692 959633